CW00507409

MEDITERRANEAN DIET COOKBOOK 6:

52 Sweets & desserts recipes.

The cookbook to conclude dinner with satisfaction. Enjoy preparing the most wanted sweets and desserts from the Mediterranean cuisine

Lily Attridge

SWEETS AND DESSERTS **8**

SWEETS AND DESSERTS

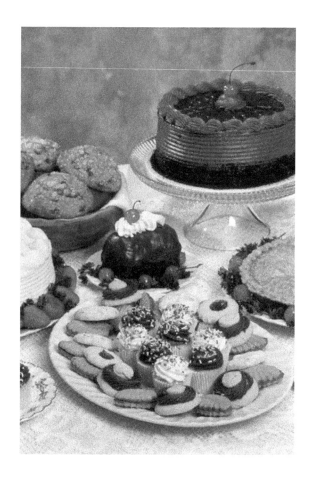

1.Stuffed Dried Figs

Preparation Time: 20 minutes
Cooking Time: 0 minutes
Servings: 4

Ingredients:

- 12 dried figs
- 2 Tbsps. thyme honey
- 2 Tbsps. sesame seeds
- 24 walnut halves

Directions:

1. Cut off the tough stalk ends of the figs.
2. Slice open each fig.
3. Stuff the fig openings with two walnut halves and close
4. Arrange the figs on a plate, drizzle with honey, and sprinkle the sesame seeds on it.
5. Serve.

Nutrition:

Calories: 110kcal
Carbs: 26
Fat: 3g,
Protein: 1g

2.Feta Cheesecake

Preparation Time: 30 minutes
Cooking Time: 90 minutes
Servings: 12

Ingredients:

- 2 cups graham cracker crumbs (about 30 crackers)
- ½ tsp ground cinnamon
- 6 tbsps. unsalted butter, melted
- ½ cup sesame seeds, toasted
- 12 ounces cream cheese, softened
- 1 cup crumbled feta cheese
- 3 large eggs
- 1 cup of sugar
- 2 cups plain yogurt
- 2 tbsps. grated lemon zest
- 1 tsp vanilla

Directions:

1. Set the oven to 350°F.
2. Mix the cracker crumbs, butter, cinnamon, and sesame seeds with a fork. Transfer the mixture to a springform pan and spread until it is even. Refrigerate.

3. In a separate bowl, mix the cream cheese and feta. With an electric mixer, beat both kinds of cheese together. Add the eggs one after the other, beating the mixture with each new addition. Add sugar, then keep beating until creamy. Mix in yogurt, vanilla, and lemon zest.

4. Bring out the refrigerated springform and spread the batter on it. Then place it in a baking pan. Fill the baking pan with water until it is halfway full.

5. Bake for about 50 minutes. Remove cheesecake and allow it to cool. Refrigerate for at least 4 hours.

6. It is done. Serve when ready.

Nutrition:

Calories: 98kcal
Carbs: 7g
Fat: 7g
Protein: 3g

3.Pear Croustade

Preparation Time: 30 minutes
Cooking Time: 60 minutes
Servings: 10
Ingredients:

- 1 cup plus 1 tbsp. all-purpose flour, divided

- 4 ½ tbsps. sugar, divided
- 1/8 tsp salt
- 6 tbsps. unsalted butter, chilled, cut into ½ inch cubes
- 1 large-sized egg, separated
- 1 / ½ tbsps. ice-cold water
- 3 firm, ripe pears (Bosc), peeled, cored, sliced into ¼ inch slices 1 tbsp. fresh lemon juice
- 1/3 tsp ground allspice
- 1 tsp anise seeds

Directions:

1. Pour 1 cup of flour, 1 ½ Tbsps. of sugar, butter, and salt into a food processor and combine the ingredients by pulsing.

2. Whisk the yolk of the egg and ice water in a separate bowl. Mix the egg mixture with the flour mixture. It will form a dough, wrap it, and set aside for an hour.

3. Set the oven to 400°F.

4. Mix the pear, sugar, leftover flour, allspice, anise seed, and lemon juice in a large bowl to make a filling.

5. Arrange the filling on the center of the dough.

6. Bake for about 40 minutes. Cool for about 15 minutes before serving.

Nutrition:

Calories: 498kcal
Carbs: 32g
Fat: 32g
Protein: 18g

4.Melomakarona

Preparation Time: 20 minutes
Cooking Time: 45 minutes
Servings: 20

Ingredients:

- 4 cups of sugar, divided
- 4 cups of water
- 1 cup plus 1 tbsp. honey, divided
- 1 (2-inch) strip orange peel, pith removed
- 1 cinnamon stick
- ½ cup extra-virgin olive oil
- ¼ cup unsalted butter,
- ¼ cup Metaxa brandy or any other brandy
- 1 tbsp. grated
- Orange zest

- ¾ cup of orange juice
- ¼ tsp baking soda
- 3 cups pastry flour
- ¾ cup fine semolina flour
- 1 ½ tsp baking powder
- 4 tsp ground cinnamon, divided
- 1 tsp ground cloves, divided
- 1 / cups finely chopped walnuts
- 1/3 cup brown sugar

Directions:

1. Mix 3 ½ cups of sugar, 1 cup honey, orange peel, cinnamon stick, and water in a pot and heat it for about 10 minutes.

2. Mix the sugar, oil, and butter for about minutes, then add the brandy, leftover honey, and zest. Then add a mixture of baking soda and orange juice. Mix thoroughly.

3. In a separate bowl, mix the pastry flour, baking powder, semolina, 2 tsp Of cinnamon, and ½ tsp. of cloves. Add the mixture to the mixer slowly. Run the mixer until the ingredients form a dough. Cover and set aside for 30 minutes.

4. Set the oven to 350°F

5. With your palms, form small oval balls from the dough. Make a total of forty balls.

6. Bake the cookie balls for 30 minutes, then drop them in the prepared syrup.

7. Create a mixture with the walnuts, leftover cinnamon, and cloves. Spread the mixture on the top of the baked cookies.

8. Serve the cookies or store them in a closed-lid container.

Nutrition:

Calories: 294kcal
Carbs: 44g
Fat: 12g
Protein: 3g

5. Loukoumades (Fried Honey Balls)

Preparation Time: 20 minutes
Cooking Time: 45 minutes
Servings: 10

Ingredients:

- 2 cups of sugar

- 1 cup of water

- 1 cup honey

- 1 ½ cups tepid water

- 1 tbsp. brown sugar

- ¼ cup of vegetable oil
- 1 tbsp. active dry yeast
- 1 ½ cups all-purpose flour, 1 cup cornstarch, ½ tsp salt
- Vegetable oil for frying
- 1 ½ cups chopped walnuts
- ¼ cup ground cinnamon

Directions:

1. Boil the sugar and water on medium heat. Add honey after 10 minutes. cool and set aside.

2. Mix the tepid water, oil, brown sugar,' and yeast in a large bowl. Allow it to sit for 10 minutes. In another bowl, mix the flour, salt, and cornstarch. With your hands mix the yeast and the flour to make a wet dough. Cover and set aside for 2 hours.

3. Fry in oil at 350°F. Use your palm to measure the sizes of the dough as they are dropped in the frying pan. Fry each batch for about 3-4 minutes.

4. Immediately the loukoumades are done frying, drop them in the prepared syrup.

5. Serve with cinnamon and walnuts.

Nutrition:

Calories: 355kcal
Carbs: 64g

Fat: 7g
Protein: 6g

6.Crème Caramel

Preparation Time: 1 hour
Cooking Time: 1 hour
Servings: 12

Ingredients:

- 5 cups of whole milk
- 2 tsp vanilla extract
- 8 large egg yolks
- 4 large-sized eggs
- 2 cups sugar, divided
- ¼ cup 0f water

Directions:

1. Preheat the oven to 350°F
2. Heat the milk on medium heat until it is scalded.
3. Mix 1 cup of sugar and eggs in a bowl and add it to the eggs.
4. With a nonstick pan on high heat, boil the water and remaining sugar. Do not stir, instead whirl the pan. When the sugar forms caramel, divide it into ramekins.

5. Divide the egg mixture into the ramekins and place in a baking pan. Add water to the pan until it is half full. Bake for 30 minutes.

6. Remove the ramekins from the baking pan, cool, then refrigerate for at least 8 hours.

7. Serve.

Nutrition:

Calories: 110kcal
Carbs: 21g
Fat: 1g
Protein: 2g

7.Galaktoboureko

Preparation Time: 30 minutes
Cooking Time: 90 minutes
Servings: 12

Ingredients:

- 4 cups sugar, divided
- 1 tbsp. fresh lemon juice
- 1 cup of water
- 1 Tbsp. plus 1 ½ tsp grated lemon zest, divided into 10 cups
- Room temperature whole milk

- 1 cup plus 2 tbsps. unsalted butter, melted and divided into 2

- Tbsps. vanilla extract

- 7 large-sized eggs

- 1 cup of fine semolina

- 1 package phyllo, thawed and at room temperature

Directions:

1. Preheat oven to 350°F

2. Mix 2 cups of sugar, lemon juice, 1 ½ tsp of lemon zest, and water. Boil over medium heat. Set aside.

3. Mix the milk, 2 Tbsps. of butter, and vanilla in a pot and put on medium heat. Remove from heat when milk is scalded

4. Mix the eggs and semolina in a bowl, then add the mixture to the scalded milk. Put the egg-milk mixture on medium heat. Stir until it forms a custard-like material.

5. Brush butter on each sheet of phyllo and arrange all over the baking pan until everywhere is covered. Spread the custard on the bottom pile phyllo

6. Arrange the buttered phyllo all over the top of the custard until every inch is covered.

7. Bake for about 40 minutes. cover the top of the

pie with all the prepared syrup. Serve.

Nutrition:

Calories: 393kcal
Carbs: 55g
Fat: 15g
Protein: 8g

8.Kourabiedes Almond Cookies

Preparation Time: 20 minutes
Cooking Time: 50 minutes
Servings: 20

Ingredients:

- 1 ½ cups unsalted butter, clarified, at room temperature 2 cups
- Confectioners' sugar, divided
- 1 large egg yolk
- 2 tbsps. brandy
- 1 1/2 tsp baking powder
- 1 tsp vanilla extract
- 5 / cups all-purpose flour, sifted
- 1 cup roasted almonds, chopped

Directions:

1. Preheat the oven to 350°F

2. Thoroughly mix butter and ½ cup of sugar in a bowl. Add in the egg after a while. Create a brandy mixture by mixing the brandy and baking powder. Add the mixture to the egg, add vanilla, then keep beating until the ingredients are properly blended

3. Add flour and almonds to make a dough.

4. Roll the dough to form crescent shapes. You should be able to get about 40 pieces. Place the pieces on a baking sheet, then bake in the oven for 25 minutes.

5. Allow the cookies to cool, then coat them with the remaining confectioner's sugar.

6. Serve.

Nutrition:

Calories: 102kcal
Carbs: 10g
Fat: 7g
Protein: 2g

9.Ekmek Kataifi

Preparation Time: 30 minutes
Cooking Time: 45 minutes
Servings: 10

Ingredients:

- 1 cup of sugar
- 1 cup of water
- 2 (2-inch) strips lemon peel, pith removed
- 1 tbsp. fresh lemon juice
- ½ cup plus 1 tbsp. unsalted butter, melted
- ½lbs. frozen kataifi pastry, thawed, at room temperature
- 2 ½ cups whole milk
- ½ tsp. ground mastiha
- 2 large eggs
- ¼ cup fine semolina
- 1 tsp. of cornstarch
- ¼ cup of sugar
- ½ cup sweetened coconut flakes
- 1 cup whipping cream
- 1 tsp. vanilla extract
- 1 tsp. powdered milk

- 3 tbsps. of confectioners' sugar
- ½ cup chopped unsalted pistachios

Directions:

1. Set the oven to 350°F. Grease the baking pan with 1. Tbsp of butter.

2. Put a pot on medium heat, then add water, sugar, lemon juice, lemon peel. Leave to boil for about 10 minutes. Reserve.

3. Untangle the kataifi, coat with the leftover butter, then place in the baking pan.

4. Mix the milk and mastiha, then place it on medium heat. Remove from heat when the milk is scalded, then cool the mixture.

5. Mix the eggs, cornstarch, semolina, and sugar in a bowl, stir thoroughly, then whisk the cooled milk mixture into the bowl.

6. Transfer the egg and milk mixture to a pot and place on heat. Wait for it to thicken like custard, then add the coconut flakes and cover it with a plastic wrap. Cool.

7. Spread the cooled custard-like material over the kataifi. Place in the refrigerator for at least 8 hours.

8. Strategically remove the kataifi from the pan with a knife. Remove it in such a way that the mold faces up.

9. Whip a cup of cream, add 1 tsp. vanilla, 1tsp. powdered milk, and 3 tbsps. Of sugar. Spread the mixture all over the custard, wait for it to harden, then flip and add the leftover cream mixture to the kataifi side.

10.   Serve.

Nutrition:

Calories: 649kcal
Carbs: 37g
Fat: 52g
Protein: 11g

10. Revani Syrup Cake

Preparation Time: 30 minutes
Cooking Time: 3 hours
Servings: 24

Ingredients:

- 1 tbsp. unsalted butter
- 2 tbsps. all-purpose flour
- 1 cup ground rusk or bread crumbs
- 1 cup fine semolina flour
- ¾ cup ground toasted almonds
- 3 tsp baking powder
- 16 large eggs
- 2 tbsps. vanilla extract
- 3 cups of sugar, divided
- 3 cups of water
- 5 (2-inch) strips lemon peel, pith removed
- 3 tbsps. fresh lemon juice
- 1 oz of brandy

Directions:

1. Preheat the oven to 350°F. Grease the baking pan with 1 Tbsp. of butter and flour.
2. Mix the rusk, almonds, semolina, baking powder in a bowl.

3. In another bowl, mix the eggs, 1 cup of sugar, vanilla, and whisk with an electric mixer for about 5 minutes. Add the semolina mixture to the eggs and stir.

4. Pour the stirred batter into the greased baking pan and place in the preheated oven.

5. With the remaining sugar, lemon peels, and water make the syrup by boiling the mixture on medium heat. Add the lemon juice after 6 minutes, then cook for 3 minutes. Remove the lemon peels and set the syrup aside.

6. After the cake is done in the oven, spread the syrup over the cake.

7. Cut the cake as you please and serve.

Nutrition:

Calories: 348kcal
Carbs: 55g
Fat: 9g
Protein: 5g

11.Almonds and Oats Pudding

Preparation Time: 10 minutes
Cooking Time: 15 minutes
Servings: 4

Ingredients:

- 1 tablespoon lemon juice
- Zest of 1 lime
- 1 and ½ cups of almond milk
- 1 teaspoon almond extract
- ½ cup oats
- 2 tablespoons stevia
- ½ cup silver almonds, chopped

Directions:

1. In a pan, combine the almond milk with the lime zest and the other ingredients, whisk, bring to a simmer and cook over medium heat for 15 minutes.
2. Divide the mix into bowls and serve cold.

Nutrition:

Calories 174
Fat 12.1
Fiber 3.2
Carbs 3.9
Protein 4.8

12.Chocolate Cups

Preparation Time: 2 hours
Cooking Time: 0 minutes
Servings: 6

Ingredients:

- ½ cup avocado oil
- 1 cup, chocolate, melted
- 1 teaspoon matcha powder
- 3 tablespoons stevia

Directions:

1. In a bowl, mix the chocolate with the oil and the rest of the ingredients, whisk well, divide into cups and keep in the freezer for 2 hours before serving.

Nutrition:

Calories 174
Fat 9.1
Fiber 2.2
Carbs 3.9
Protein 2.8

13. Mango Bowls

Preparation Time: 30 minutes
Cooking Time: 0 minutes
Servings: 4

Ingredients:

- 3 cups mango, cut into medium chunks
- ½ cup of coconut water
- ¼ cup stevia
- 1 teaspoon vanilla extract

Directions:

1. In a blender, combine the mango with the rest of the ingredients, pulse well, divide into bowls and serve cold.

Nutrition:

Calories 122
Fat 4
Fiber 5.3
Carbs 6.6
Protein 4.5

14.Cocoa and Pears Cream

Preparation Time: 10 minutes
Cooking Time: 0 minutes
Servings: 4

Ingredients:

- 2 cups heavy creamy
- 1/3 cup stevia
- ¾ cup cocoa powder
- 6 ounces dark chocolate, chopped
- Zest of 1 lemon
- 2 pears, chopped

Directions:

1. In a blender, combine the cream with the stevia and the rest of the ingredients, pulse well, divide into cups and serve cold.

Nutrition:

Calories 172
Fat 5.6
Fiber 3.5
Carbs 7.6
Protein 4

15.Pineapple Pudding

Preparation Time: 10 minutes
Cooking Time: 40minutes
Servings: 4

Ingredients:

- 3 cups almond flour
- ¼ cup olive oil
- 1 teaspoon vanilla extract
- 2 and ¼ cups stevia
- 3 eggs, whisked
- 1 and ¼ cup natural apple sauce
- 2 teaspoons baking powder
- 1 and ¼ cups of almond milk
- 2 cups pineapple, chopped
- Cooking spray

Directions:

1. In a bowl, combine the almond flour with the oil and the rest of the ingredients except the cooking spray and stir well.

2. Grease a cake pan with the cooking spray, pour the pudding mix inside, introduce in the oven and bake at 370 degrees F for 40 minutes.

3. Serve the pudding cold.

Nutrition:

Calories 223
Fat 8.1
Fiber 3.4
Carbs 7.6
Protein 3.4

16.Lime Vanilla Fudge

Preparation Time: 3 hours
Cooking Time: 0 minutes
Servings: 6

Ingredients:

- 1/3 cup cashew butter

- 5 tablespoons lime juice

- ½ teaspoon lime zest, grated

- 1 tablespoons stevia

Directions:

1. In a bowl, mix the cashew butter with the other ingredients and whisk well.

2. Line a muffin tray with parchment paper, scoop 1 tablespoon of lime fudge mix in each of the muffin tins and keep in the freezer for 3 hours before serving.

Nutrition:

Calories 200

Fat 4.5
Fiber 3.4
Carbs 13.5
Protein 5

17.Mixed Berries Stew

Preparation Time: 10 minutes
Cooking Time: 15 minutes
Servings: 6

Ingredients:

- Zest of 1 lemon, grated
- Juice of 1 lemon
- ½ pint blueberries
- 1-pint strawberries halved
- 2 cups of water
- 2 tablespoons stevia

Directions:

1. In a pan, combine the berries with the water, stevia and the other ingredients, bring to a simmer, cook over medium heat for 15 minutes, divide into bowls and serve cold.

Nutrition:

Calories 172
Fat 7
Fiber 3.4
Carbs 8
Protein 2.3

18.Orange and Apricots Cake

Preparation Time: 10 minutes
Cooking Time: 20 minutes
Servings: 8

Ingredients:

- ¾ cup stevia
- 2 cups almond flour
- ¼ cup olive oil
- ½ cup almond milk
- 1 teaspoon baking powder
- 2 eggs
- ½ teaspoon vanilla extract
- Juice and zest of 2 oranges
- 2 cups apricots, chopped

Directions:

1. In a bowl, mix the stevia with the flour and the rest of the ingredients, whisk and pour into a cake pan lined with parchment paper.

2. Introduce in the oven at 375 degrees F, bake for 20 minutes, cool down, slice and serve.

Nutrition:

Calories 221
Fat 8.3

Fiber 3.4
Carbs 14.5
Protein 5

19.Blueberry Cake

Preparation Time: 10 minutes
Cooking Time: 30 minutes
Servings: 6

Ingredients:

- 2 cups almond flour
- 3 cups blueberries
- 1 cup walnuts, chopped
- 3 tablespoons stevia
- 1 teaspoon vanilla extract
- 2 eggs, whisked
- 2 tablespoons avocado oil
- 1 teaspoon baking powder
- Cooking spray

Directions:

1. In a bowl, combine the flour with the blueberries, walnuts and the other ingredients except for the cooking spray, and stir well.

2. Grease a cake pan with the cooking spray, pour the cake mix inside, introduce everything in the oven at 350 degrees F and bake for 30 minutes.

3. Cool the cake down, slice and serve.

Nutrition:

Calories 225
Fat 9
Fiber 4.5
Carbs 10.2
Protein 4.5

20.Blueberry Yogurt Mousse

Preparation Time: 30 minutes
Cooking Time: 0 minutes
Servings: 4

Ingredients:

- 2 cups Greek yogurt

- ¼ cup stevia

- ¾ cup heavy cream

- 2 cups blueberries

Directions:

1. In a blender, combine the yogurt with the other ingredients, pulse well, divide into cups and keep in the fridge for 30 minutes before serving.

Nutrition:

Calories 141
Fat 4.7
Fiber 4.7
Carbs 8.3
Protein 0.8

21.Almond Peaches Mix

Preparation Time: 10 minutes
Cooking Time: 10 minutes
Servings: 4

Ingredients:

- 1/3 cup almonds, toasted
- 1/3 cup pistachios, toasted
- 1 teaspoon mint, chopped
- ½ cup of coconut water
- 1 teaspoon lemon zest, grated
- 4 peaches, halved
- 2 tablespoons stevia

Directions:

1. In a pan, combine the peaches with the stevia and the rest of the ingredients, simmer over medium heat for 10 minutes, divide into bowls and serve cold.

Nutrition:

Calories 135
Fat 4.1
Fiber 3.8
Carbs 4.1
Protein 2.3

22.Walnuts Cake

Preparation Time: 10 minutes
Cooking Time: 40 minutes
Servings: 4

Ingredients:

- ½ pound walnuts, minced
- Zest of 1 orange, grated
- 1 and ¼ cups stevia
- eggs whisked
- 1 teaspoon almond extract
- 1 and ½ cup of almond flour
- 1 teaspoon baking soda

Directions:

1. In a bowl, combine the walnuts with the orange zest and the other ingredients, whisk well and pour into a cake pan lined with parchment paper.
2. Introduce in the oven at 350 degrees F, bake for 40 minutes, cool down, slice and serve.

Nutrition:

Calories 205
Fat 14.1
Fiber 7.8
Carbs 9.1
Protein 3.4

23.Hazelnut Pudding

Preparation Time: 10 minutes
Cooking Time: 40 minutes
Servings: 8

Ingredients:

- 2 and ¼ cups almond flour
- 3 tablespoons hazelnuts, chopped
- 5 eggs, whisked
- 1 cup stevia
- 1 and 1/3 cups Greek yogurt
- 1 teaspoon baking powder
- 1 teaspoon vanilla extract

Directions:

1. In a bowl, combine the flour with the hazelnuts and the other ingredients, whisk well, and pour into a cake pan lined with parchment paper,
2. Introduce in the oven at 350 degrees F, bake for 30 minutes, cool down, slice and serve.

Nutrition:

Calories 178
Fat 8.4
Fiber 8.2
Carbs 11.5
Protein 1.4

24.Cinnamon Banana and Semolina Pudding

Preparation Time: 5 minutes
Cooking Time: 7 minutes
Servings: 6

Ingredients:

- 2 cups semolina, ground
- 1 cup olive oil
- 4 cups hot water
- 2 bananas, peeled and chopped
- 1 teaspoon cinnamon powder
- 4 tablespoons stevia

Directions:

1. Heat a pan with the oil over medium-high heat, add the semolina and brown it for 3 minutes stirring often.
2. Add the water and the rest of the ingredients except the cinnamon, stir, and simmer for 4 minutes more.

Divide into bowls, sprinkle the cinnamon on top and serve.

Nutrition:

Calories 162
Fat 8,
Fiber 4.2
Carbs 4.3
Protein 8.4

25.Banana Shake Bowls

Preparation Time: 5 minutes
Cooking Time: 0 minutes
Servings: 4

Ingredients:

- 4 medium bananas, peeled
- 1 avocado, peeled, pitted and mashed
- ¾ cup almond milk
- ½ teaspoon vanilla extract

Directions:

1. In a blender, combine the bananas with the avocado and the other ingredients, pulse, divide into bowls and keep in the fridge until serving.

Nutrition:

Calories 185
Fat 4.3
Fiber 4
Carbs 6
Protein 6.45

26.Cold Lemon Squares

Preparation Time: 30 minutes
Cooking Time: 0 minutes
Servings: 4

Ingredients:

- 1 cup avocado oil+ a drizzle
- 2 bananas, peeled and chopped
- 1 tablespoon honey
- ¼ cup lemon juice
- A pinch of lemon zest, grated

Directions:

1. In your food processor, mix the bananas with the rest of the ingredients, pulse well and spread on the bottom of a pan greased with a drizzle of oil.
2. Introduce in the fridge for 30 minutes, slice into squares and serve.

Nutrition:

Calories 136
Fat 11.2
Fiber 0.2
Carbs 7
Protein 1.1

27.Blackberry and Apples Cobbler

Preparation Time: 10 minutes
Cooking Time: 30 minutes
Servings: 6

Ingredients:

- ¾ cup stevia
- 6 cups blackberries
- ¼ cup apples, cored and cubed
- ¼ teaspoon baking powder
- 1 tablespoon lime juice
- ½ cup almond flour
- ½ cup of water
- 3 and ½ tablespoon avocado oil
- Cooking spray

Directions:

1. In a bowl, mix the berries with half of the stevia and lemon juice, sprinkle some flour all over, whisk and pour into a baking dish greased with cooking spray.

2. In another bowl, mix flour with the rest of the sugar, baking powder, the water, and the oil, and stir the whole thing with your hands.

3. Spread over the berries, introduce in the oven at 375 degrees F and bake for 30 minutes.

4. Serve warm.

Nutrition:

Calories 221
Fat 6.3
Fiber 3.3
Carbs 6
Protein 9

28.Black Tea Cake

Preparation Time: 10 minutes
Cooking Time: 35 minutes
Servings: 8

Ingredients:

- 6 tablespoons black tea powder
- 2 cups almond milk, warmed up
- 1 cup avocado oil
- 2 cups stevia
- 4 eggs
- 2 teaspoons vanilla extract
- 3 and ½ cups almond flour
- 1 teaspoon baking soda
- 3 teaspoons baking powder

Directions:

1. In a bowl, combine the almond milk with the oil, stevia and the rest of the ingredients and whisk well.

2. Pour this into a cake pan lined with parchment paper, introduce in the oven at 350 degrees F and bake for 35 minutes.

3. Leave the cake to cool down, slice and serve.

Nutrition:

Calories 200
Fat 6.4
Fiber 4
Carbs 6.5
Protein 5.4

29. Green Tea and Vanilla Cream

Preparation Time: 2 hours
Cooking Time: 0 minutes
Servings: 4

Ingredients:

- 14 ounces almond milk, hot
- 2 tablespoons green tea powder
- 14 ounces heavy cream
- 3 tablespoons stevia
- 1 teaspoon vanilla extract

- 1 teaspoon gelatin powder

Directions:

1. In a bowl, combine the almond milk with the green tea powder and the rest of the ingredients, whisk well, cool down, divide into cups and keep in the fridge for 2 hours before serving.

Nutrition:

Calories 120
Fat 3
Fiber 3
Carbs 7
Protein 4

30.Figs Pie

Preparation Time: 10 minutes
Cooking Time: 1 hour
Servings: 8

Ingredients:

- ½ cup stevia
- 6 figs, cut into quarters
- ½ teaspoon vanilla extract
- 1 cup almond flour
- 4 eggs, whisked

Directions:

1. Spread the figs on the bottom of a springform pan lined with parchment paper.

2. In a bowl, combine the other ingredients, whisk and pour over the figs,

3. Bake at 375 digress F for 1 hour, flip the pie upside down when it's done and serve.

Nutrition:

Calories 200
Fat 4.4
Fiber 3
Carbs 7.6
Protein 8

31.Cherry Cream

Preparation Time: 2 hours
Cooking Time: 0 minutes
Servings: 4

Ingredients:

- 2 cups cherries, pitted and chopped

- 1 cup almond milk

- ½ cup whipping cream

- 3 eggs, whisked

- 1/3 cup stevia

- 1 teaspoon lemon juice

- ½ teaspoon vanilla extract

Directions:

1. In your food processor, combine the cherries with the milk and the rest of the ingredients, pulse well, divide into cups and keep in the fridge for 2 hours before serving.

Nutrition:

Calories 200
Fat 4.5
Fiber 3.3
Carbs 5.6
Protein 3.4

32.Strawberries Cream

Preparation Time: 10 minutes
Cooking Time: 20 minutes
Servings: 4

Ingredients:

- ½ cup stevia

- 2 pounds strawberries, chopped

- 1 cup almond milk

- Zest of 1 lemon, grated

- ½ cup heavy cream

- 3 egg yolks, whisked

Directions:

1. Heat a pan with the milk over medium-high heat, add the stevia and the rest of the ingredients, whisk well, simmer for 20 minutes, divide into cups and serve cold.

Nutrition:

Calories 152
Fat 4.4
Fiber 5.5
Carbs 5.1
Protein 0.8

33.Apples and Plum Cake

Preparation Time: 10 minutes
Cooking Time: 40 minutes
Servings: 4

Ingredients:

- 7 ounces almond flour
- 1 egg, whisked
- 5 tablespoons stevia
- 3 ounces warm almond milk
- 2 pounds plums, pitted and cut into quarters
- 2 apples, cored and chopped
- Zest of 1 lemon, grated
- 1 teaspoon baking powder

Directions:

1. In a bowl, mix the almond milk with the egg, stevia, and the rest of the ingredients except the cooking spray and whisk well.

2. Grease a cake pan with the oil, pour the cake mix inside, introduce in the oven and bake at 350 degrees F for 40 minutes.

3. Cool down, slice and serve.

Nutrition:

Calories 209
Fat 6.4
Fiber 6
Carbs 8
Protein 6.6

34.Cinnamon Chickpeas Cookies

Preparation Time: 10 minutes
Cooking Time: 20 minutes
Servings: 12

Ingredients:

- 1 cup canned chickpeas, drained, rinsed and mashed
- 2 cups almond flour
- 1 teaspoon cinnamon powder
- 1 teaspoon baking powder
- 1 cup avocado oil
- ½ cup stevia
- 1 egg, whisked
- 2 teaspoons almond extract
- 1 cup raisins
- 1 cup coconut, unsweetened and shredded

Directions:

1. In a bowl, combine the chickpeas with the flour, cinnamon, and the other ingredients, and whisk well until you obtain a dough.

2. Scoop tablespoons of dough on a baking sheet lined with parchment paper, introduce them in the oven at 350 degrees F and bake for 20 minutes.

3. Leave them to cool down for a few minutes and serve.

Nutrition:

Calories 200
Fat 4.5
Fiber 3.4
Carbs 9.5
Protein 2.4

35.Cocoa Brownies

Preparation Time: 10 minutes
Cooking Time: 20 minutes
Servings: 8

Ingredients:

- 30 ounces canned lentils, rinsed and drained
- 1 tablespoon honey
- 1 banana, peeled and chopped
- ½ teaspoon baking soda
- 4 tablespoons almond butter
- 2 tablespoons cocoa powder
- Cooking spray

Directions:

1. In a food processor, combine the lentils with the honey and the other ingredients except for the cooking spray and pulse well.

2. Pour this into a pan greased with cooking spray, spread evenly, introduce in the oven at 375 degrees F and bake for 20 minutes.

3. Cut the brownies and serve cold.

Nutrition:

Calories 200
Fat 4.5
Fiber 2.4
Carbs 8.7
Protein 4.3

36.Cardamom Almond Cream

Preparation Time: 30 minutes
Cooking Time: 0 minutes
Servings: 4

Ingredients:

- Juice of 1 lime
- ½ cup stevia
- 1 and ½ cups of water
- 3 cups almond milk
- ½ cup honey
- 2 teaspoons cardamom, ground
- 1 teaspoon rose water
- 1 teaspoon vanilla extract

Directions:

1. In a blender, combine the almond milk with the cardamom and the rest of the ingredients, pulse well, divide into cups and keep in the fridge for 30 minutes before serving.

Nutrition:

Calories 283
Fat 11.8
Fiber 0.3
Carbs 4.7
Protein 7.1

37.Banana Cinnamon Cupcakes

Preparation Time: 10 minutes
Cooking Time: 20 minutes
Servings: 4

Ingredients:

4 tablespoons avocado oil

4 eggs

½ cup of orange juice

2 teaspoons cinnamon powder

1 teaspoon vanilla extract

2 bananas, peeled and chopped

¾ cup almond flour

½ teaspoon baking powder

Cooking spray

Directions:

In a bowl, combine the oil with the eggs, orange juice and the other ingredients except for the cooking spray, whisk well, pour in a cupcake pan greased with the cooking spray, introduce in the oven at 350 degrees F and bake for 20 minutes.

Cool the cupcakes down and serve.

Nutrition:

Calories 142
Fat 5.8

Fiber 4.2
Carbs 5.7
Protein 1.6

38.Rhubarb and Apple Cream

Preparation Time: 10 minutes
Cooking Time: 0 minutes
Servings: 6

Ingredients:

- 3 cups rhubarb, chopped

- 1 and ½ cups stevia

- 2 eggs, whisked

- ½ teaspoon nutmeg, ground

- 1 tablespoon avocado oil

- 1/3 cup almond milk

Directions:

1. In a blender, combine the rhubarb with the stevia and the rest of the ingredients, pulse well, divide into cups and serve cold.

Nutrition:

Calories 200
Fat 5.2
Fiber 3.4
Carbs 7.6
Protein 2.5

39.Almond Rice Dessert

Preparation Time: 10 minutes
Cooking Time: 20 minutes
Servings: 4

Ingredients:

- 1 cup white rice
- 2 cups almond milk
- 1 cup almonds, chopped
- ½ cup stevia
- 1 tablespoon cinnamon powder
- ½ cup pomegranate seeds

Directions:

1. In a pot, mix the rice with the milk and stevia, bring it to a simmer and cook for 20 minutes, stirring often.
2. Add the rest of the ingredients, stir, divide into bowls and serve.

Nutrition:

Calories 234
Fat 9.5
Fiber 3.4
Carbs 12.4
Protein 6.5

40.Peach Sorbet

Preparation Time: 2 hours
Cooking Time: 10 minutes
Servings: 4

Ingredients:

- 2 cups apple juice

- 1 cup stevia

- 2 tablespoons lemon zest, grated

- 2 pounds peaches, pitted and quartered

Directions:

1. Heat a pan over medium heat, add the apple juice and the rest of the ingredients, simmer for 10 minutes, transfer to a blender, pulse, divide into cups and keep in the freezer for 2 hours before serving.

Nutrition:

Calories 182
Fat 5.4
Fiber 3.4
Carbs 12
Protein 5.4

41.Cranberries and Pears Pie

Preparation Time: 10 minutes
Cooking Time: 40 minutes
Servings: 4

Ingredients:

- 2 cup cranberries
- 3 cups pears, cubed
- A drizzle of olive oil
- 1 cup stevia
- 1/3 cup almond flour
- 1 cup rolled oats
- ¼ avocado oil

Directions:

1. In a bowl, mix the cranberries with the pears and the other ingredients except for the olive oil and the oats, and stir well.

2. Grease a cake pan with a drizzle of olive oil, pour the pears mix inside, sprinkle the oats all over and bake at 350 degrees F for 40 minutes.

3. Cool the mix down, and serve.

Nutrition:

Calories 172
Fat 3.4
Fiber 4.3
Carbs 11.5
Protein 4.5

42.Lemon Cream

Preparation Time: 1 hour
Cooking Time: 10 minutes
Servings: 6

Ingredients:

- 2 eggs, whisked
- 1 and ¼ cup stevia
- 10 tablespoons avocado oil
- 1 cup heavy cream
- Juice of 2 lemons
- Zest of 2 lemons, grated

Directions:

1. In a pan, combine the cream with the lemon juice and the other ingredients, whisk well, cook for 10 minutes, divide into cups and keep in the fridge for 1 hour before serving.

Nutrition:

Calories 200
Fat 8.5
Fiber 4.5
Carbs 8.6
Protein 4.5

43.Blueberries Stew

Preparation Time: 10 minutes
Cooking Time: 10 minutes
Servings: 4

Ingredients:

- 2 cups blueberries
- 3 tablespoons stevia
- 1 and ½ cups pure apple juice
- 1 teaspoon vanilla extract

Directions:

1. In a pan, combine the blueberries with stevia and the other ingredients, bring to a simmer and cook over medium-low heat for 10 minutes.
2. Divide into cups and serve cold.

Nutrition:

Calories 192
Fat 5.4
Fiber 3.4
Carbs 9.4
Protein 4.5

44.Mandarin Cream

Preparation Time: 20 minutes
Cooking Time: 0 minutes
Servings: 8

Ingredients:

- 2 mandarins, peeled and cut into segments
- Juice of 2 mandarins
- 2 tablespoons stevia
- 4 eggs, whisked
- ¾ cup stevia
- ¾ cup almonds, ground

Directions:

1. In a blender, combine the mandarins with the mandarins juice and the other ingredients, whisk well, divide into cups and keep in the fridge for 20 minutes before serving.

Nutrition:

Calories 106
Fat 3.4
Fiber 0
Carbs 2.4
Protein 4

45.Creamy Mint Strawberry Mix

Preparation Time: 10 minutes
Cooking Time: 30 minutes
Servings: 6

Ingredients:

- Cooking spray
- ¼ cup stevia
- 1 and ½ cup of almond flour
- 1 teaspoon baking powder
- 1 cup almond milk
- 1 egg, whisked
- 2 cups strawberries, sliced
- 1 tablespoon mint, chopped
- 1 teaspoon lime zest, grated
- ½ cup whipping cream

Directions:

1. In a bowl, combine the almond with the strawberries, mint and the other ingredients except for the cooking spray and whisk well.

2. Grease 6 ramekins with the cooking spray, pour the strawberry mix inside, introduce in the oven and bake at 350 degrees F for 30 minutes.

3. Cooldown and serve.

Nutrition:

Calories 200
Fat 6.3
Fiber 2
Carbs 6.5
Protein 8

46.Vanilla Cake

Preparation Time: 10 minutes
Cooking Time: 25 minutes
Servings: 10

Ingredients:

- 3 cups almond flour
- 3 teaspoons baking powder
- 1 cup olive oil
- 1 and ½ cup of almond milk
- 1 and 2/3 cup stevia
- 2 cups of water
- 1 tablespoon lime juice
- 2 teaspoons vanilla extract
- Cooking spray

Directions:

1. In a bowl, mix the almond flour with the baking

powder, the oil and the rest of the ingredients except the cooking spray and whisk well.

2. Pour the mix into a cake pan greased with the cooking spray, introduce in the oven and bake at 370 degrees F for 25 minutes.

3. Leave the cake to cool down, cut and serve!

Nutrition:

Calories 200
Fat 7.6
Fiber 2.5
Carbs 5.5
Protein 4.5

47.Pumpkin Cream

Preparation Time: 5 minutes
Cooking Time: 5 minutes
Servings: 2

Ingredients:

- 2 cups canned pumpkin flesh
- 2 tablespoons stevia
- 1 teaspoon vanilla extract
- 2 tablespoons water
- A pinch of pumpkin spice

Directions:

1. In a pan, combine the pumpkin flesh with the other ingredients, simmer for 5 minutes, divide into cups and serve cold.

Nutrition:

Calories 192
Fat 3.4
Fiber 4.5
Carbs 7.6
Protein 3.5

48.Chia and Berries Smoothie Bowl

Preparation Time: 5 minutes
Cooking Time: 0 minutes
Servings: 2

Ingredients:

- 1 and ½ cup of almond milk
- 1 cup blackberries
- ¼ cup strawberries, chopped
- 1 and ½ tablespoons chia seeds
- 1 teaspoon cinnamon powder

Directions:

1. In a blender, combine the blackberries with the strawberries and the rest of the ingredients, pulse well, divide into small bowls and serve cold.

Nutrition:

Calories 182
Fat 3.4
Fiber 3.4
Carbs 8.4
Protein 3

49.Minty Coconut Cream

Preparation Time: 4 minutes
Cooking Time: 0 minutes
Servings: 2

Ingredients:

- 1 banana, peeled
- 2 cups coconut flesh, shredded
- 3 tablespoons mint, chopped
- 1 and ½ cups of coconut water
- 2 tablespoons stevia
- ½ avocado pitted and peeled

Directions:

In a blender, combine the coconut with the banana and the rest of the ingredients, pulse well, divide into cups and serve cold.

Nutrition:

Calories 193
Fat 5.4
Fiber 3.4
Carbs 7.6
Protein 3

50.Watermelon Cream

Preparation Time: 15 minutes
Cooking Time: 0 minutes
Servings: 2

Ingredients:

- 1 pound watermelon, peeled and chopped
- 1 teaspoon vanilla extract
- 1 cup heavy cream
- 1 teaspoon lime juice
- 2 tablespoons stevia

Directions:

1. In a blender, combine the watermelon with the cream and the rest of the ingredients, pulse well, divide into cups and keep in the fridge for 15 minutes before serving.

Nutrition:

Calories 122
Fat 5.7
Fiber 3.2
Carbs 5.3
Protein 0.4

51.Grapes Stew

Preparation Time: 10 minutes
Cooking Time: 10 minutes
Servings: 4

Ingredients:

- 2/3 cup stevia
- 1 tablespoon olive oil
- 1/3 cup coconut water
- 1 teaspoon vanilla extract
- 1 teaspoon lemon zest, grated
- 2 cup red grapes, halved

Directions:

1. Heat a pan with the water over medium heat, add the oil, stevia and the rest of the ingredients, toss, simmer for 10 minutes, divide into cups and serve.

52.Cocoa Sweet Cherry Cream

Preparation Time: 2 hours
Cooking Time: 0 minutes
Servings: 4

Ingredients:

- ½ cup of cocoa powder
- ¾ cup red cherry jam
- ¼ cup stevia
- 2 cups of water
- 1 pound cherries, pitted and halved

Directions:

1. In a blender, mix the cherries with the water and the rest of the ingredients, pulse well, divide into cups and keep in the fridge for 2 hours before serving.

Nutrition:

Calories 162
Fat 3.4
Fiber 2.4
Carbs 5
Protein 1

53.Apple Couscous Pudding

Preparation Time: 10 minutes
Cooking Time: 25 minutes
Servings: 4

Ingredients:

- ½ cup couscous
- 1 and ½ cups of milk
- ¼ cup apple, cored and chopped
- 3 tablespoons stevia
- ½ teaspoon rose water
- 1 tablespoon orange zest, grated

Directions:

1. Heat a pan with the milk over medium heat, add the couscous and the rest of the ingredients, whisk, simmer for 25 minutes, divide into bowls and serve.

Nutrition:

Calories 150
Fat 4.5
Fiber 5.5
Carbs 7.5
Protein 4

54.Ricotta Ramekins

Preparation Time: 10 minutes
Cooking Time: 1 hour
Servings: 4

Ingredients:

- 6 eggs, whisked
- 1 and ½ pounds ricotta cheese, soft
- ½ pound stevia
- 1 teaspoon vanilla extract
- ½ teaspoon baking powder
- Cooking spray

Directions:

1. In a bowl, mix the eggs with the ricotta and the other ingredients except for the cooking spray and whisk well.
2. Grease 4 ramekins with the cooking spray, pour the ricotta cream in each and bake at 360 degrees F for 1 hour.
3. Serve cold.

Nutrition:

Calories 180
Fat 5.3
Fiber 5.4
Carbs 11.5

Protein 4

55.Papaya Cream

Preparation Time: 10 minutes
Cooking Time: 0 minutes
Servings: 2

Ingredients:

- 1 cup papaya, peeled and chopped
- 1 cup heavy cream
- 1 tablespoon stevia
- ½ teaspoon vanilla extract

Directions:

1. In a blender, combine the cream with the papaya and the other ingredients, pulse well, divide into cups and serve cold.

Nutrition:

Calories 182
Fat 3.1
Fiber 2.3
Carbs 3.5
Protein 2